# The Survival Medicine Guide

## How to Treat and Prevent Injuries, Illnesses, and Other Medical Emergencies When Help is Not an Option

## MADISON PARKS

# Table of Contents

# INTRODUCTION

Welcome to the World of Survival Medicine. In the realm of survival, where unforeseen challenges lurk around every corner, understanding the principles of survival medicine becomes paramount. This introduction serves as your gateway into a world where medical emergencies unfold in unpredictable environments, far removed from the comforts of traditional healthcare settings. Survival medicine is not merely a set of skills; it is a mindset and a comprehensive approach to addressing injuries, illnesses, and emergencies when conventional help is not readily available.

## Understanding the Importance of Survival Medicine

In the broader landscape of healthcare, survival medicine carves its niche as a specialized discipline that prepares individuals to navigate the unique challenges posed by adverse conditions. Unlike routine medical care, survival medicine focuses on providing essential and immediate medical assistance in environments where access to professional healthcare may be compromised or nonexistent. It delves into the core principles of assessing, stabilizing, and addressing health issues with limited resources, making it an indispensable skill set for anyone venturing into the unpredictable terrains of the great outdoors or facing unforeseen circumstances.

## The Unique Challenges of Medical Emergencies in Survival Situations

Survival situations introduce a myriad of challenges that necessitate a different set of responses from traditional healthcare practices. The lack of immediate access to hospitals, medical professionals, and even basic supplies amplifies the complexity of medical emergencies. Survival medicine grapples with factors such as extreme weather conditions, limited resources, and the need for improvisation in the absence of modern medical facilities. Understanding these unique challenges is crucial for developing the adaptability and resilience required to address health crises in austere environments.

# Why Should I Read This Book?

Assessing the Relevance of Survival Medicine in Everyday Life is the first step in recognizing the broader applicability of survival medicine beyond extreme scenarios. While initially perceived as a skillset reserved for adventurers and outdoor enthusiasts, the relevance of survival medicine extends to everyday life. Emergencies can happen anywhere, from the comfort of your home to a routine commute, and being equipped with the knowledge to handle them can make a significant difference.

## Assessing the Relevance of Survival Medicine in Everyday Life

Survival medicine is not exclusive to those venturing into the wilderness; it holds substantial relevance in everyday life. Accidents, sudden illnesses, or unexpected emergencies can occur in various settings, from the workplace to family outings. The ability to provide immediate and effective medical assistance becomes a valuable asset in ensuring the well-being of yourself and those around you. Understanding the basics of survival medicine empowers individuals to respond confidently to unexpected health challenges, fostering a sense of preparedness in day-to-day activities.

## Building a Foundation for Medical Preparedness

This book lays the foundation for medical preparedness by offering a comprehensive guide to building the necessary skills and knowledge. It goes beyond addressing emergencies and seeks to instill a proactive mindset towards health. By delving into the principles of survival medicine, readers embark on a journey of self-reliance, understanding that preparedness is not solely about responding to crises but also about preventing them where possible. The chapters ahead unfold as a roadmap for cultivating a robust foundation in medical preparedness, encompassing both theoretical knowledge and practical skills.

In conclusion, this guide serves as a beacon in the realm of survival medicine. As you delve into the subsequent chapters, you will embark on a transformative journey, gaining insights into the intricacies of survival medicine and discovering the empowerment that comes with being prepared for the unexpected. Whether you are an outdoor enthusiast, a parent, or an individual navigating the challenges of daily life, the principles outlined within these pages will become a valuable companion on your quest for medical readiness. Welcome to a world where knowledge becomes a lifeline, and preparedness becomes a way of life.

# Chapter 1

# Assessing and Responding to Immediate Threats

In the crucible of emergency situations, the ability to swiftly assess and respond to immediate threats is a cornerstone of survival medicine. Recognizing life-threatening emergencies is the first critical skill explored in this chapter. Amidst chaos and uncertainty, understanding the distinction between minor issues and those that demand urgent attention becomes paramount. This skill extends beyond the purview of healthcare professionals, empowering individuals from all walks of life to identify situations where immediate action is crucial.

## Recognizing Life-Threatening Emergencies

Life-threatening emergencies manifest in various forms, from cardiac events to severe trauma. The chapter navigates through the intricacies of recognizing critical signs and symptoms, providing readers with a comprehensive understanding of the diverse array of emergencies they might encounter. A focus on early detection and assessment lays the groundwork for effective response, highlighting the significance of remaining vigilant in assessing the well-being of oneself and others in high-stress situations.

## Identifying Critical Signs and Symptoms

Within the tapestry of medical emergencies, certain signs and symptoms act as red flags, indicating the severity of the situation. This section explores the nuanced art of identifying these critical indicators. From altered levels of consciousness to abnormal vital signs, readers gain insights into the subtle cues that could denote an impending crisis. Armed with this knowledge, individuals are better equipped to make rapid, informed decisions in the face of uncertainty, ultimately improving the chances of positive outcomes in emergencies.

# Prioritizing Actions in High-Stress Situations

High-stress situations often accompany emergencies, clouding judgment and creating an environment where split-second decisions matter. This part of the chapter focuses on the psychological aspects of responding to immediate threats. It delves into the importance of maintaining a calm and collected demeanor, emphasizing the need for a systematic approach to prioritize actions. Readers gain an understanding of how effective decision-making under pressure is not just a skill but a mindset cultivated through knowledge and preparation.

# Basic First Aid Techniques

With the foundation of recognizing and prioritizing in place, the chapter seamlessly transitions into basic first aid techniques. This section acts as a hands-on guide, equipping individuals with the fundamental skills needed to address a variety of medical emergencies. From minor injuries to more severe incidents, the emphasis is on providing immediate assistance with the resources available. Basic first aid becomes a bridge between recognizing a problem and implementing a solution, offering a tangible way to intervene before professional help arrives.

## Wound Care and Bandaging

Wound care stands as a cornerstone of basic first aid, and this section delves into the intricacies of managing injuries effectively. Readers learn the principles of wound assessment, understanding the different types of wounds and their corresponding treatments. The art of bandaging takes center stage, exploring the various techniques for securing dressings and immobilizing injured areas. Practical insights into wound care not only enhance immediate response capabilities but also contribute to long-term recovery outcomes.

## Handling Fractures and Sprains

Fractures and sprains pose unique challenges, requiring a nuanced approach for effective management. This segment of the chapter unravels the complexities of recognizing and addressing skeletal injuries. Readers gain insights into differentiating between fractures and sprains, understanding the importance of immobilization, and exploring improvised techniques for creating splints. By the end, individuals are equipped to provide crucial support in situations where professional medical assistance may be delayed or unavailable.

## Managing Burns and Scalds

Burns and scalds represent another category of injuries demanding immediate attention. This part of the chapter delves into the intricacies of burn management, from assessing the severity of burns to implementing appropriate first aid measures. Understanding the different degrees of burns and the corresponding treatment approaches becomes crucial knowledge for anyone navigating survival scenarios. Practical tips on cooling burns, applying dressings, and monitoring for complications round out this comprehensive guide to managing thermal injuries effectively.

In essence, This Chapter serves as a foundational pillar in the edifice of survival medicine. Readers are not only introduced to the critical skills of recognizing and assessing immediate threats but are also guided through practical techniques for responding to a spectrum of emergencies. From understanding subtle signs to executing hands-on first aid procedures, this chapter lays the groundwork for a well-rounded approach to medical preparedness in the face of life-threatening situations.

# Chapter 2

# Essential Medical Supplies for Your Survival Kit

Creating a Comprehensive Medical Kit is the bedrock of medical preparedness, and this chapter serves as a guide to assembling a toolkit tailored for survival scenarios. The intricacies of choosing and packing medical supplies are explored, ensuring that individuals are equipped to handle a spectrum of health issues in environments where professional healthcare is not readily accessible.

## Creating a Comprehensive Medical Kit

Building a medical kit for survival requires a thoughtful and strategic approach. Readers delve into the essentials of selecting appropriate containers, considering factors such as size, portability, and durability. The chapter explores the spectrum of medical supplies needed, ranging from the basics like bandages and antiseptics to more specialized items for trauma care and emergencies. Practical tips on organizing the kit for easy access under stress lay the foundation for a well-structured and efficient medical arsenal.

## Medications and Pain Relief

Understanding the role of medications in a survival kit is paramount. This section navigates the complexities of choosing and storing medications effectively. Readers gain insights into common over-the-counter medications, prescription drugs, and their potential uses in different scenarios. Pain relief becomes a focal point, exploring both pharmaceutical and natural alternatives. The chapter emphasizes the importance of considering individual medical needs and potential allergic reactions when curating the medication component of the survival kit.

## Bandages, Dressings, and Sterilization Tools

Bandages and dressings are the frontline defenses against injuries, making them crucial components of any survival kit. This segment delves into the different types of bandages and dressings, their applications, and considerations for selecting the most appropriate ones for various injuries. Sterilization tools take center stage, with discussions on antiseptics, disinfectants, and improvised sterilization techniques. Understanding the importance of maintaining a sterile environment when managing wounds contributes significantly to positive health outcomes.

## Tools for Minor Surgical Procedures

In survival scenarios, the need may arise for minor surgical procedures that go beyond basic first aid. This part of the chapter explores the inclusion of tools for such situations. Readers are introduced to the concept of minor surgical kits, including instruments for wound exploration, suturing, and other procedures. Practical insights into using these tools in austere environments underscore the importance of being prepared for a spectrum of medical interventions beyond the scope of conventional first aid.

# Understanding Expiry Dates and Rotation

The effectiveness of a survival kit hinges on the viability of its contents. This section tackles the critical aspect of understanding expiry dates and rotation. Readers gain insights into the lifespan of different medical supplies, medications, and the factors that can affect their shelf life. The chapter emphasizes the need for a systematic approach to regularly check and rotate items within the kit, ensuring that, when the time comes, the supplies are not only present but also in optimal condition for use.

# Maintaining and Updating Your Medical Supplies

A comprehensive medical kit is a dynamic entity that requires regular attention. This part of the chapter delves into the principles of maintaining and updating supplies. From routine checks to addressing wear and tear, readers gain practical tips on ensuring the longevity and reliability of their medical kit. The chapter underscores the importance of staying informed about advancements in medical preparedness, prompting individuals to update their kits to reflect evolving best practices and recommendations.

## Adapting Your Kit to Different Survival Scenarios

Survival scenarios vary widely, and a one-size-fits-all approach to medical preparedness may fall short. This segment explores the art of adapting the medical kit to different survival scenarios. From wilderness excursions to urban emergencies, readers gain insights into tailoring their kits to the specific challenges posed by diverse environments. Practical considerations, such as climate, potential hazards, and anticipated medical needs, guide individuals in creating versatile and adaptable medical kits capable of addressing a spectrum of survival situations.

In essence, This Chapter unfolds as a guide to crafting a lifeline in the form of a well-curated medical kit. From the basics of bandaging to the intricacies of medications and surgical tools, readers embark on a journey of understanding the essential components necessary for effective medical preparedness. The chapter's holistic approach ensures that individuals not only assemble a comprehensive survival kit but also cultivate the skills needed to maintain and adapt it, fostering a sense of confidence in the face of health challenges in unpredictable environments.

# Chapter 3

## Dealing with Common Infections and Illnesses

In the unpredictable landscapes of survival scenarios, the ability to deal with common infections and illnesses becomes a linchpin of medical preparedness. This chapter navigates the intricacies of infection prevention strategies and the nuanced approach to treating ailments when professional medical assistance is not readily available.

## Infection Prevention Strategies

Preventing infections in survival environments is not only about responding to crises but also adopting a proactive stance towards health. This section explores the foundational principles of infection prevention, emphasizing the significance of maintaining personal hygiene and creating a clean environment. Readers gain insights into the importance of routine checks for cuts and abrasions, as these seemingly minor issues can escalate into major infections in austere settings. The chapter underscores the interconnectedness of infection prevention strategies with overall well-being, fostering a holistic approach to health in challenging conditions.

## Hygiene Practices in Survival Environments

Hygiene practices take center stage as a critical aspect of infection prevention. This part of the chapter delves into the practicalities of maintaining personal hygiene in survival environments where resources may be limited. From improvised soap alternatives to strategies for waste disposal, readers gain practical insights into cultivating habits that minimize the risk of infections. The chapter underscores the importance of integrating hygiene practices into daily routines, transforming them from isolated tasks into integral components of a broader health-focused mindset.

## Safe Water Sourcing and Purification

Access to safe water is a fundamental requirement for survival, and ensuring its safety becomes paramount in preventing waterborne infections. This segment explores the intricacies of safe water sourcing and purification. Readers gain insights into identifying potential water sources, understanding the risks associated with different environments, and employing effective purification methods. The chapter demystifies the process of water purification, empowering individuals to make informed decisions about the safety of the water they consume, a pivotal aspect of infection prevention in survival scenarios.

## Treating Common Ailments

The chapter seamlessly transitions from prevention to treatment, addressing the nuances of handling common ailments when professional medical help is not readily available. This section equips readers with the knowledge needed to navigate a spectrum of health issues that may arise in survival settings.

## Respiratory Infections and Illnesses

Respiratory infections pose a significant threat in confined or crowded survival environments. This part of the chapter delves into the intricacies of recognizing and managing respiratory issues. From understanding the symptoms of common colds to addressing more severe respiratory infections, readers gain insights into providing effective care. Practical tips on creating improvised cough syrups and maintaining air quality in enclosed spaces underscore the resourcefulness required in managing respiratory ailments when conventional treatments are not accessible.

## Gastrointestinal Issues and Foodborne Illnesses

Survival scenarios often involve reliance on limited food resources, and gastrointestinal issues can quickly become prevalent. This section explores the complexities of treating common digestive ailments and foodborne illnesses. Readers gain practical knowledge on identifying symptoms, implementing basic dietary modifications, and understanding the importance of food safety in preventing infections. The chapter emphasizes the need for caution in food preparation and storage, highlighting how preventive measures can significantly reduce the risk of gastrointestinal issues in survival environments.

In essence, Chapter 3 becomes a comprehensive guide to navigating the intricate terrain of infections and illnesses in survival scenarios. From the proactive stance of infection prevention to the hands-on approach of treating common ailments, readers embark on a journey of understanding the interconnectedness of health practices in austere environments. The chapter not only equips individuals with the knowledge to prevent and address infections but also cultivates a mindset of adaptability and resourcefulness, essential qualities for thriving in challenging health conditions.

# Chapter 4

# Emergency Dental Care in Survival Situations

## Dental Emergency Preparedness

In the realm of survival medicine, the importance of dental emergency preparedness often takes a back seat, yet the significance becomes glaringly evident when faced with toothaches, infections, or dental traumas in austere environments. This chapter unravels the complexities of being prepared for dental emergencies, providing a comprehensive guide on how to navigate and address unforeseen dental issues when professional care is not readily available.

## Recognizing Dental Issues and Infections

The first step in effective emergency dental care is the ability to recognize dental issues and infections promptly. This section delves into the nuanced signs and symptoms that indicate potential problems, ranging from tooth decay and abscesses to gum infections. Readers gain insights into the importance of regular dental checks even in survival scenarios, as early detection becomes pivotal in preventing minor dental concerns from escalating into major issues. The chapter emphasizes the interconnectedness of oral health with overall well-being in challenging environments.

## Improvised Dental Tools and Techniques

In survival situations, access to professional dental tools may be nonexistent. This part of the chapter explores the art of improvisation, guiding readers through the creation of improvised dental tools and techniques. From crafting toothbrushes from natural materials to developing makeshift floss, individuals learn resourceful strategies to maintain oral hygiene. Practical insights into improvising dental mirrors and explorers highlight the adaptability required in addressing dental concerns when conventional tools are not at hand.

# Pain Management and Temporary Solutions

Dental pain can be debilitating, and effective pain management becomes a critical aspect of emergency dental care. This segment delves into the nuances of alleviating dental pain using both conventional and improvised methods. Readers gain practical knowledge on utilizing over-the-counter pain relievers, as well as exploring natural remedies to manage discomfort. Temporary solutions for common dental issues, such as loose fillings or lost crowns, become integral components of the survival toolkit, offering relief until more permanent solutions can be implemented.

# Addressing Dental Trauma in the Absence of Professional Care

Dental trauma, ranging from chipped teeth to more severe injuries, presents unique challenges in survival scenarios. This section becomes a guide to addressing dental trauma when professional care is not readily available. Readers gain insights into the immediate steps to take when faced with injuries such as knocked-out teeth or fractures. The chapter explores the improvisation of splints and methods for stabilizing dental injuries temporarily. Practical tips on managing bleeding and preventing infections in the aftermath of dental trauma become essential knowledge for individuals navigating survival environments.

In essence, Chapter 4 unfolds as a crucial resource in the survival medicine guide, shining a spotlight on an often-overlooked aspect of healthcare. Dental emergencies, though not always life-threatening, can significantly impact an individual's well-being and ability to function optimally. By delving into the intricacies of dental emergency preparedness, recognizing issues promptly, and offering practical solutions for pain management and trauma, this chapter equips readers with the knowledge and skills needed to address dental concerns effectively when professional care is out of reach.

# Chapter 5

# Mental Health and Well-being in Survival Scenarios

In the intricate tapestry of survival scenarios, mental health and well-being weave through the very fabric of resilience and adaptability. This chapter delves into the profound impact of psychological health on survival, recognizing the importance of addressing stress, isolation, and mental health challenges in high-stress environments.

## Recognizing and Managing Stress

Stress is an inevitable companion in survival situations, and understanding how to recognize and manage it becomes paramount for overall well-being. This section explores the nuanced signs of stress, ranging from heightened anxiety to fatigue. Readers gain insights into effective stress management techniques, including mindfulness exercises, deep breathing, and the power of positive thinking. The chapter underscores the interconnectedness of mental and physical health, emphasizing that managing stress is not only a psychological endeavor but a holistic approach to thriving in challenging circumstances.

## Coping Strategies in Isolation

Isolation, whether self-imposed or a consequence of survival scenarios, presents unique challenges to mental health. This part of the chapter unravels coping strategies tailored to the realities of isolation. From maintaining routines to fostering connections with nature, readers gain practical insights into cultivating a resilient mindset when faced with prolonged periods of aloneness. The chapter emphasizes the importance of self-awareness and adaptability, recognizing that effective coping strategies evolve with the evolving dynamics of isolation in survival scenarios.

## Building Resilience in High-Stress Environments

Resilience becomes a beacon of strength in high-stress environments, and this section guides readers through the process of building and nurturing resilience. Practical tips on embracing challenges as opportunities for growth, developing problem-solving skills, and fostering a positive mindset become integral components of resilience in survival situations. The chapter navigates the nuances of bouncing back from setbacks, reinforcing the idea that resilience is not just an innate quality but a skill that can be cultivated through knowledge and intentional practices.

## Psychological First Aid

Just as physical first aid is crucial in emergencies, psychological first aid plays a pivotal role in addressing mental health challenges. This segment explores the principles of psychological first aid, providing readers with a guide on how to offer immediate support to individuals experiencing distress. From active listening to providing reassurance, readers gain insights into the nuances of offering empathetic and effective psychological first aid. The chapter underscores the importance of fostering a supportive environment, recognizing that mental well-being is often a collective endeavor in survival scenarios.

# Providing Support to Others in Stressful Situations

Survival scenarios often involve navigating challenges as a group, and providing support to others in stressful situations becomes a collective responsibility. This section delves into the dynamics of offering support to fellow survivors, recognizing the power of community in mitigating stress and promoting mental well-being. Practical tips on effective communication, building trust, and creating a supportive atmosphere contribute to the development of a cohesive and resilient group dynamic. The chapter emphasizes that in survival scenarios, the mental well-being of individuals is interwoven with the well-being of the group.

# Recognizing Signs of Mental Health Challenges

The chapter concludes by shedding light on the importance of recognizing signs of mental health challenges. From anxiety disorders to post-traumatic stress, readers gain insights into the nuanced indicators that may signal the presence of mental health issues. The chapter emphasizes the destigmatization of mental health discussions in survival scenarios, fostering an environment where individuals feel comfortable seeking and offering support. Recognizing signs early becomes a pivotal step in addressing mental health challenges proactively and cultivating an atmosphere of understanding and compassion.

In essence, Chapter 5 emerges as a cornerstone in the survival medicine guide, acknowledging the profound impact of mental health on overall well-being. From stress management to building resilience and offering psychological first aid, readers embark on a journey of understanding the interconnectedness of mental and physical health in survival scenarios. This chapter not only equips individuals with the knowledge to navigate the complexities of psychological challenges but also fosters a mindset of collective support and resilience, essential qualities for thriving in high-stress environments.

# Conclusion

## Reflecting on Your Preparedness Journey

As we bring this comprehensive survival medicine guide to a close, it's essential to embark on a journey of reflection. Reflecting on your preparedness journey is not just a retrospective exercise but a crucial step in fortifying your readiness for future challenges. Consider the knowledge gained, the skills honed, and the mindset cultivated throughout the exploration of survival medicine. It's a moment to acknowledge the empowerment that comes from being proactive about your health and well-being in unpredictable environments. This reflection becomes a compass guiding you forward, ensuring that the lessons learned become a resilient foundation for whatever lies ahead.

## Continuous Learning and Skill Development

The journey of preparedness is an ongoing one, and the knowledge acquired is a catalyst for continuous learning and skill development. In the realm of survival medicine, staying stagnant is not an option. This section encourages individuals to embrace the ethos of lifelong learning, seeking out new information, and staying abreast of advancements in medical preparedness. Whether it's exploring emerging treatments, refining first aid techniques, or delving into the intricacies of improvised tools, the commitment to continuous learning ensures that your survival medicine skills remain sharp and adaptable.

## Staying Proactive in Maintaining Medical Readiness

Maintaining medical readiness is not a passive endeavor; it requires proactive engagement and are highlighted as essential steps. Staying proactive involves periodic reviews of your knowledge and skills, perhaps engaging in refresher courses or seeking additional certifications to enhance your medical preparedness arsenal.

Moreover, staying proactive in maintaining medical readiness extends beyond individual efforts. Consider fostering a sense of collective preparedness within your community or group. This could involve sharing knowledge, conducting training sessions, or collaborating on the development of emergency response plans. By contributing to a network of prepared individuals, you not only enhance your own readiness but also contribute to the resilience of the broader community.

Reflecting on the experiences shared throughout this guide, it becomes evident that preparedness is not solely about having the right supplies or knowing specific medical techniques. It is a holistic approach that encompasses mental resilience, adaptability, and a commitment to continuous improvement. Staying proactive in maintaining medical readiness is a dynamic process that requires dedication, curiosity, and a willingness to adapt to evolving circumstances.

In conclusion, the journey through the chapters of this survival medicine guide has been a voyage into the heart of preparedness. From assessing and responding to immediate threats to navigating the complexities of mental health in survival scenarios, each chapter has contributed to a comprehensive understanding of medical preparedness. As you reflect on your preparedness journey, recognize the transformation from a passive recipient of information to an active participant in your own well-being.

Continuous learning and skill development are the pillars that support this journey. The landscape of medicine is ever-evolving, and by embracing a mindset of lifelong learning, you position yourself not only as a survivor but as a resilient individual capable of adapting to a myriad of challenges. This guide serves as a foundation, but the journey doesn't end here; it extends into the realm of ongoing discovery and mastery.

Staying proactive in maintaining medical readiness is the culmination of reflection, learning, and a commitment to readiness. It is an acknowledgment that preparedness is not a destination but a continual process of growth and adaptation. As you navigate the uncertainties of the future, let this guide be a compass, and let your journey be marked by a dedication to your well-being and that of those around you. The chapters explored have illuminated the path; now, it is up to you to walk it with resilience, knowledge, and a readiness to face whatever challenges may come.